in
the
news™

PANDEMICS

EPIDEMICS IN
A SHRINKING WORLD

Miriam Segall

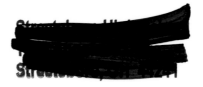

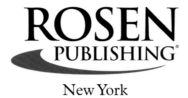

ROSEN
PUBLISHING®

New York

To my parents

Published in 2007 by The Rosen Publishing Group, Inc.
29 East 21st Street, New York, NY 10010

First Edition

Library of Congress Cataloging-in-Publication Data

Segall, Miriam.
Pandemics: epidemics in a shrinking world / Miriam Segall.—1st ed.
    p. cm.—(In the news)
Includes bibliographical references.
ISBN-13: 978-1-4042-0975-6
ISBN-10: 1-4042-0975-1 (lib. bdg.)
1. Epidemics—Juvenile literature. 2. Communicable diseases—Juvenile literature. I. Title.
RA653.5.S44 2007
614.4—dc22

                                                                    2006024437

Manufactured in the United States of America

On the Cover: Clockwise from top left: A health worker in southwest China culls chickens to halt the spread of avian flu; doctors examine a man in Indonesia suspected of having avian flu; duck farms in Bulgaria hope to avoid contact with influenza; and Los Angeles Department of Health worker Emily Moore administers an influenza vaccine.

contents

What Is a Pandemic?

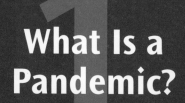

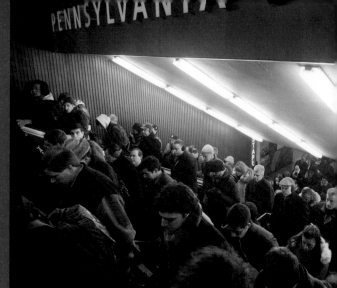

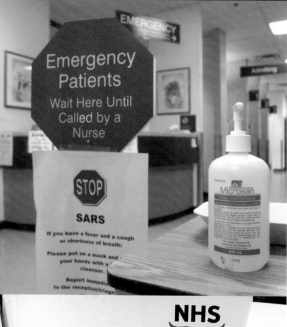

When most people think about disease and the spread of germs, they think about isolated outbreaks, or epidemics, of disease. Epidemics occur within confined populations and geographical areas, while pandemics are epidemics that have spread across the globe. Pandemics have the potential to spread disease far and wide. Pandemics spread quickly and have the potential to affect millions of people.

According to the World Health Organization (WHO), several factors must be present

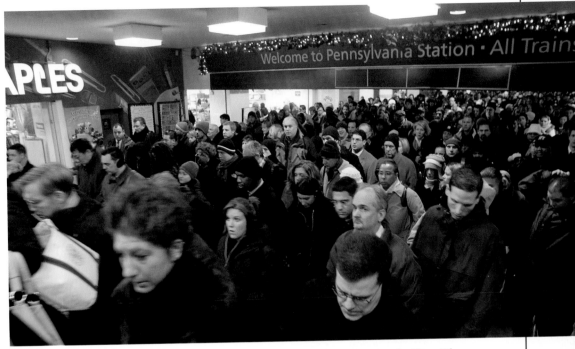

Commuters exit Penn Station during rush hour in New York City. The airborne transmission of virus particles in metropolitan transit hubs concerns public health officials.

for an epidemic to be considered a pandemic. First, the disease must have never appeared before within a population; second, the agent that carries the disease—like a fly, bacteria, air, or water—infects one person, causing serious illness; and last, the disease spreads easily among humans.

Pandemics in America

The first major pandemic on U.S. soil occurred nearly a century ago, beginning in 1918, when the influenza virus killed more than 600,000 people, forcing scientists and doctors to take a hard look at methods to control the spread of disease. This horrific outbreak that took Americans by surprise became known as the Spanish flu. Curiously, nearly a century later, scientists now predict that the next great pandemic threat America will likely face will be another, different strain of the influenza virus. Given the increase in the U.S. population, if another influenza virus spreads at the same rate as the Spanish flu did, more than 1.4 million people would perish while hundreds of thousands more would be weakened from the disease.

> *In little more than a month, 195,000 Americans died, making influenza the nation's greatest killer of all time. When Americans celebrated the end of World War I in the streets of New York in 1918, they did so with masks over their faces.*

In the fall of 1918, the Spanish flu emerged like a sleeping giant, largely killing not infants and the elderly, as influenza usually does, but young people in the prime of their lives. When the virus was at its worst, the mortality rate skyrocketed, especially in congested cities. More than 11,000 people died in Philadelphia in October 1918. One day in New York City brought with it 851 influenza deaths. In little more than a month, 195,000 Americans died, making influenza the nation's greatest killer of all time. When Americans celebrated the end of World War I

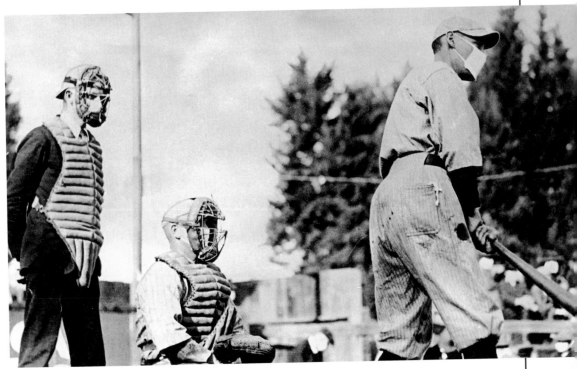

In this photograph from 1918, a baseball player is seen wearing a mask for protection against the transmission of influenza germs during the Spanish flu epidemic.

in the streets in 1918, they did so with masks over their faces.

In the fall of 1918, an Ocala, Florida, man traveled to Jacksonville for a carpentry job. Jacksonville was inundated with the flu at the time, and despite a citywide quarantine and the use of gauze masks, the man contracted the flu. Eager to return to his hometown and family, he slipped past the quarantine and caught a train back home, taking the virus with him. Within days of his return, he had infected his family, and was bedridden with his son. The man recovered, but others were not as fortunate.

In 1919, eight-year-old Carl Lindner shared a room in the Marion County hospital with his five-year-old cousin, Philip Townsend. Both had come down with the flu. When Philip recovered, he asked the nurses where his cousin was. The only answer the nurses could give was that Carl had already gone home. They did not know how to tell the child that his cousin was dead. Within three weeks, Carl's father and maternal grandfather also died from the disease.

The city of Jacksonville was stricken with influenza, which its population had never experienced. The people of Jacksonville had no natural immunity to the disease. The flu infected the visiting carpenter, who then spread it to his family, thus introducing the flu to a new population that could then spread it to many other people. It's like a chain reaction, or a series of cascading dominos. If the links aren't broken, or if the dominos keep falling, then the result is perpetual motion, or a continuing spread of the disease.

These stories accurately describe the beginnings of a pandemic that would eventually kill 25 million people around the world in just six months. Even though these stories are almost a century old, they still have the power to make people concerned about the future and about preparing for the possibility of another influenza pandemic.

Distinctions Between Pandemics and Epidemics

Besides the size of the region and the number of people affected, there are other distinct differences between pandemics and epidemics. WHO defines an epidemic as "an outbreak of a contagious disease that spreads quickly and affects many people." Epidemics are classified into several different types based upon how they begin and the way they are transmitted between humans. That is because epidemics can involve being exposed once, a few times, or a great many times to the disease-carrying agent—whether it's air, water, feces, or flies, to name but a few. Epidemics can also be restricted to one small area (an outbreak) or happen in a much larger one, like the population of a city, state, or country.

For an epidemic to become a pandemic, the spread of infectious disease must be global or at least present in a very large area. In other words, all pandemics are epidemics, but an epidemic can only be called a pandemic if it spreads around the world. Not all epidemics grow beyond a small population, so they are not all classified as pandemics.

It's also important to remember that a disease or condition is not a pandemic simply because it is widespread or kills a large number of people; it must also be infectious. Therefore, cancer, even though it is responsible for many deaths around the world every year, is not a pandemic. On the other hand, the HIV virus that produces AIDS is considered a pandemic because it spreads from one person to the next by means of infection. Heart disease, which is the number-one killer in the United States, is also not considered a pandemic.

Stages of a Pandemic

The Centers for Disease Control and Prevention (CDC) divides the stages of a pandemic into three general categories. The first is known as the interpandemic period, when the disease is detected in new populations. The second is called the pandemic alert period, when the disease has just begun to spread from one person to another. The third is the pandemic period, when the disease is transmitted throughout the general population.

The CDC further divides these three periods into five specific stages. The following section examines the influenza virus and divides it into these five stages.

Interpandemic Period

- **Phase 1:** No new influenza virus subtypes have been detected in humans. An influenza virus subtype that has caused human infection may be present in animals. If it is present in animals, the risk of human infection or disease is considered to be low.

- **Phase 2:** No new influenza virus subtypes have been detected in humans. However, a circulating animal influenza virus subtype poses a substantial risk of human disease.

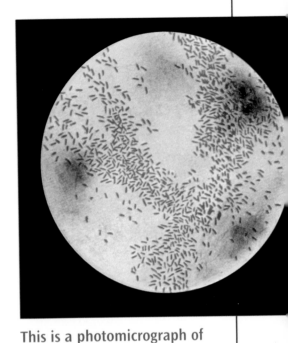

This is a photomicrograph of *Haemophilus influenzae*, circa 1947, the bacterium thought to be the cause of the 1918 influenza outbreak.

Pandemic Alert Period

- **Phase 3:** Human infection(s) with a new subtype but no human-to-human spread, or in rare instances have spread because of close contact.
- **Phase 4:** Small cluster(s) with limited human-to-human transmission but spread is highly localized, suggesting that the virus is not well adapted to humans.
- **Phase 5:** Larger cluster(s) but human-to-human spread still localized, suggesting that the virus is becoming increasingly better adapted to humans but may not yet be fully transmissible. (There is a substantial pandemic risk at this stage.)

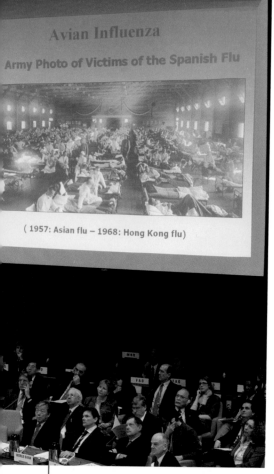

(1957: Asian flu – 1968: Hong Kong flu)

WHO executives are reminded of influenza horrors by this projection of a U.S. Army photo taken during the 1918 outbreak.

Pandemic Period

- **Phase 6:** A full-blown pandemic with increased and sustained transmission among the general population.

It is important to understand what the stages of a pandemic are because it allows government and private agencies to have a universal method for discussing pandemic threats and planning for them more effectively. Understanding the course a pandemic will take will help reduce panic and allow for prevention measures to be put into place. It is useful to have step-by-step guidelines about what to do in order to most efficiently combat the onset of a global disease outbreak.

The following chapters will examine various pandemics throughout history, what diseases still pose a global threat to humans, and what we can do to prevent or minimize the effects of a pandemic.

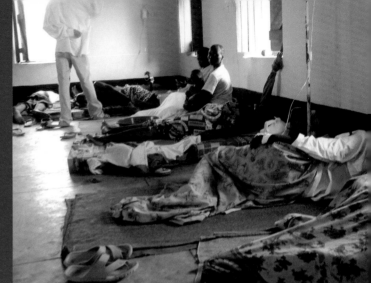

Pandemics Throughout History

2

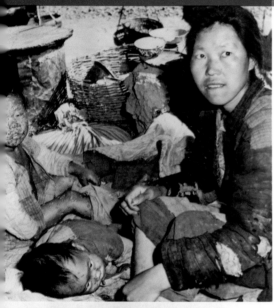

During the Middle Ages, hundreds of thousands of men, women, and children died in every country in fourteenth-century Europe, struck down by an epidemic of incurable plague that was so deadly it became known as the Black Death.

Not since the sixth century had such an epidemic attacked Europe. Carried by rats and the fleas that infested them, the disease spread from Asia to cities and towns along the ports of the Black Sea. The plague took two forms. Bubonic plague was seen in

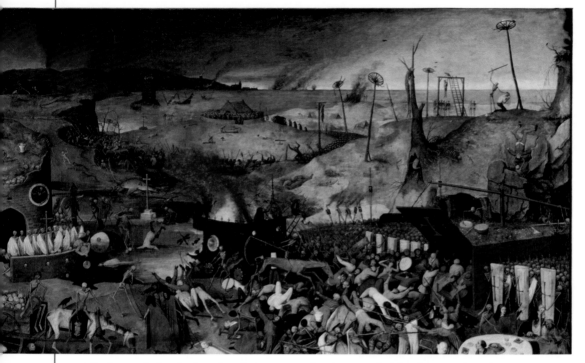

Victims of the bubonic plague are the focus of this sixteenth-century painting by Pieter Bruegel the Elder called *The Triumph of Death*.

the swellings, or buboes, that swelled the lymph nodes at the neck, armpit, or groin. When pneumonic plague affected the lungs, victims choked on their own blood.

False Hope

Doctors did what they could, but the plague was unstoppable. Even the most expert physicians could do little more than help strengthen people's resolve and build morale. Some recommended the burning of aromatic woods and herbs; others suggested special diets, courses of bleeding, new postures for sleeping, and other remedies. The wealthy attempted making medicine from gold and pearls. The terrible truth is that nothing slowed the spread of the disease. Flight was the best option, but if one could not flee, then all that remained was resignation and prayer.

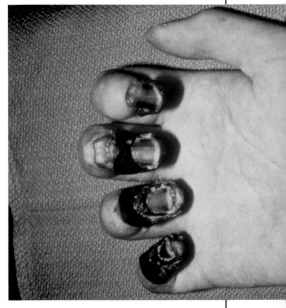

In this photograph, a plague victim shows one of its manifestations: tissues that have succumbed to gangrene. This was one reason why the disease was called the Black Death.

Pandemics have always been a part of history. Diseases such as typhus, smallpox, cholera, and influenza have wreaked havoc upon the world for more than two millennia. All one has to do is look closely at the words of the noted nursery rhyme "Ring Around the Rosie" to find clues about one of the most famous pandemics, the Black Plague. Many historians believe that the last two lines, "A-tish-shoo, a-tish-shoo, we all fall down," refer to how victims collapsed as a result of the plague's symptoms.

Ancient Pandemics

The first recognized pandemic occurred in 430 BC, as the Peloponnesian War (431–404 BC) raged between the

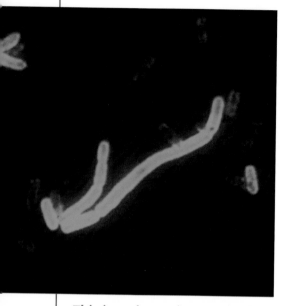

This is a photomicrograph of the bacterium *Yersinia pestis*, the organism believed to have caused the bubonic plague.

city-states Athens and Sparta for twenty-seven years. During that time, a plague killed a quarter of the population of Athens in four years, weakening its ability to fight and spurring Sparta to victory. For many years, the exact cause of the plague was unknown.

In January 2006, however, an article published in *Scientific American* reported that researchers from the University of Athens had analyzed teeth recovered from a mass grave underneath Athens, and confirmed the presence of salmonella, the bacteria responsible for typhoid fever. This disease, which is transmitted by contaminated food or water, causes fever, rash, and diarrhea. These symptoms closely matched accounts of the terrible plague by the famous Greek writer Thucydides.

In 541 BC, the Plague of Justinian made its first appearance in Egypt. According to the Byzantine-era writer Procopius, this plague killed 10,000 people a day at its height and perhaps 40 percent of the inhabitants of the city of Constantinople. Before its end, the disease had eliminated a quarter of the population of the eastern

Mediterranean region. Many centuries later, scientists proved that the Plague of Justinian was most likely the first recorded outbreak of bubonic plague, which would become far more significant centuries later during the Middle Ages.

Pandemics of the Middle Ages

Whenever the words "plague" and "pandemic" are mentioned, it's a good bet that people think about the Black Plague of the Middle Ages. This is because this disease killed more than thirty million people in Europe within six years, beginning in 1348. At the time, this figure represented a quarter of the world's total population, with more than half of the deaths occurring in affected urban areas. The bacteria *Yersinia pestis* caused the Black Plague.

Whenever the words "plague" and "pandemic" are mentioned, it's a good bet that people think about the Black Plague of the Middle Ages. This is because this disease killed more than thirty million people in Europe within six years, beginning in 1348.

Depending on what kind of plague type it is—pneumonic, which is spread in the air; septicemic, where the plague infects the bloodstream; or bubonic—the disease can be transmitted by fleas, from person to person, or by rats. Bubonic plague was the most commonly seen form during the height of the pandemic,

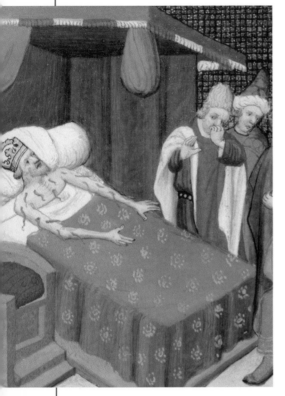

The plague was the inspiration of works of art and literature, including *The Decameron*, a medieval history book. This detail was taken from a fifteenth-century version.

with typical features including swelling in the groin and armpits, which would then ooze pus and blood, followed by skin damage in the form of dark blotches. Victims would die between four and seven days after infection. Other symptoms included fever of 101 to 105 degrees Fahrenheit (38–41 degrees Celsius), headaches, aching joints, nausea and vomiting, and a general feeling of weakness.

As it turned out, that malaise was not just limited to the effects of disease, but to the effects on European society, too. The Great Mortality, as writers at the time called it, changed Europe's social structure and greatly affected the Catholic Church, which was the most prominent religious institution of the time, as well as segregated lepers and Jews, who were believed to be agents of disease. The Black Plague also inspired great literature in the form of the Italian writer Giovanni Boccaccio. He lived through the plague as it spread through Florence, Italy, in 1348, and the experience led him to write a book, *The Decameron*, a story of seven men and three women who escape the disease by fleeing to a villa outside the city.

Although evidence suggests that the disease causing the Black Plague probably returned to Europe every generation, it finally disappeared outright in the eighteenth century, giving way to different diseases that caused a host of other problems.

Other Pandemics

Typhoid fever is sometimes confused with typhus, which refers to several diseases caused by another kind of bacteria called rickettsia. Because it has a tendency to spread widely under conditions of poor hygiene, including prison or refugee camps, among the homeless, and in armies in the field, it is sometimes called "camp fever" because of its pattern of flaring up in times of strife. Though it first emerged during the Crusades in the twelfth century, the disease

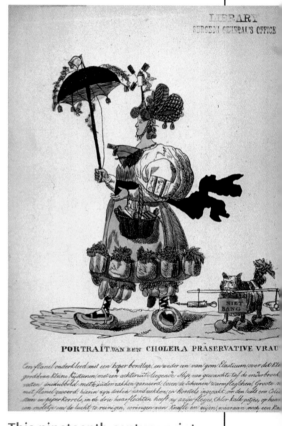

PORTRAIT van een CHOLERA PRÄSERVATIVE VRAU

This nineteenth-century print shows some of the precautions that people during that period took against cholera, including strapping hot-water bottles to their feet to prevent fever.

had great impact by killing tens of thousands in Spain in 1489, in the Balkans in 1542, and in Russia in 1812.

Even though cholera cannot spread from person to person, it has still had devastating consequences on several populations around the globe in the last two centuries, making it the most widespread pandemic to date. Cholera is considered extremely dangerous because the bacteria that causes it, *Vibrio cholerae*, gets into the water system and contaminates the water supply. As a result, thousands of people can die simply by drinking water. In a series of pandemics beginning in 1816 and ending in 1866, cholera spread from India to Europe, Russia, the Middle East, and North America, killing hundreds of thousands of people in its wake. Later instances of cholera in the 1960s led to many deaths in Bangladesh, India, and in the former Soviet Union.

Although scientists now understand what caused most of the pandemics throughout history, some remain elusive. In the sixteenth century, a disease called English Sweat swept through the United Kingdom. The onset of the disease's symptoms—cold shivers, heart palpitations, and massive outpouring of sweat—was rapid and sudden, with death taking place within hours. By 1551, English Sweat had disappeared just as mysteriously as it had begun. Even though there were many investigations into what may have caused the disease, nothing was ever discovered.

3 Modern Pandemics

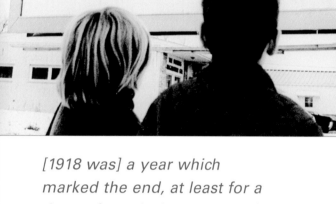

HONG KONG FLU IS UNAMERICAN!

Catch Something Made in the U.S

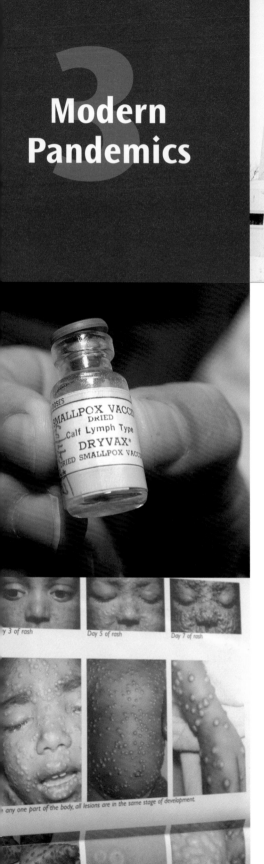

SMALLPOX VACC
DRIED
Calf Lymph Type
DRYVAX®
DRIED SMALLPOX VACC

y 3 of rash   Day 5 of rash   Day 7 of rash

any one part of the body, all lesions are in the same stage of development.

[1918 was] a year which marked the end, at least for a time, of man's destruction of man; unfortunately a year in which developed a most fatal infectious disease causing the death of hundreds of thousands of human beings. Medical science for four and one-half years devoted itself to putting men on the firing line and keeping them there. Now it must turn . . . to combating the greatest enemy of all—infectious disease.

—Journal of the American Medical Association, *1918*

The twentieth century was no stranger to the onset of pandemics.

Cholera and typhus, as well as typhoid fever, continued to ravage populations in many countries, as another lethal disease called smallpox also made its presence known. Smallpox was first thought to be a form of the Antonine plague, which killed a quarter of those infected, and up to five million between AD 165 and 180. The smallpox virus, characterized by facial pimples that can fill up with pus and become painful, potentially fatal blisters, was responsible for an estimated 300 million to 500 million deaths in the twentieth century. But thanks to the efforts of scientists going back to the eighteenth century, a vaccine against the virus was developed that finally proved successful by 1977, when the last known case of smallpox was reported.

Influenza

Most diseases, especially viruses, cannot be contained as successfully as smallpox was. That is because small changes in a virus's genetic makeup can speed its ability to infect a greater number of people. The best example of this is how a simple case of the flu led to the most lethal pandemic of the twentieth century.

The symptoms of influenza are easy to recognize. They include chills, fever, a runny nose, sore throat, coughing, and all-over body aches. Influenza is different from the common cold because the flu is caused by a

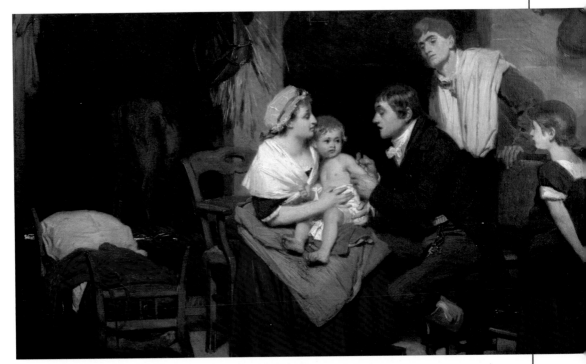

Edward Jenner, the British doctor responsible for discovering the vaccination for smallpox, is depicted in this French nineteenth-century painting.

different virus that produces symptoms that are more severe and unpleasant. The flu also infects people seasonally, which leads to long lines at hospitals and clinics to obtain a vaccine against the most recent strain of the disease. Because the flu can spread so rapidly, it can easily become a pandemic, which has happened many times throughout the 1900s.

The first and worst pandemic was the Spanish flu. It first appeared on March 11, 1918, at a U.S. Army training camp in Fort Riley, Kansas. By noon, more than 100 soldiers were sent to the camp's hospital to be treated

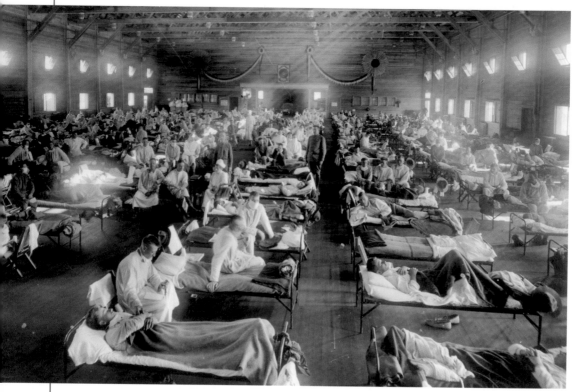

The crowded infirmary hospital at Fort Riley, Kansas, is shown in this photograph from 1918 during the midst of the worst influenza outbreak in United States history.

for flu-like symptoms. By week's end, that number jumped to 500. And by October of that year, the disease had spread across the entire United States (with more than 195,000 Americans already ill that month).

Meanwhile, the Spanish flu was quickly becoming a pandemic. It had appeared on nearly every continent by the end of 1918, its spread made more immediate by the invasion of Europe during World War I. Although the exact number of people who were infected or died has not been fully established, some estimates claim that almost 500 million people around the world suffered from the Spanish flu, and between 25 and 50 million died from it—most within six months. By early 1920, the disease had completely disappeared, vanishing almost as quickly as it had begun.

Despite its quick arrival and disappearance, the Spanish flu had a devastating impact around the world. In the United Kingdom, more than 150,000 people died, making a significant psychological and emotional impact on the nation. British doctors tried everything they could to hold back the spread of the disease, from the medieval practice of bleeding patients and administering oxygen, to developing new vaccines. But only one stopgap measure, transfusing the blood of recovered patients to those still infected with the flu, was met with success.

In the United States, the problems and conflicts associated with the outbreak were no different. Everyone was impacted—the Spanish flu infected all victims, whether they were rich or poor, old or young, and notable or unknown. Among its more well-known victims were silent screen star Harold Lockwood, U.S. Army General John Pershing, Hollywood and stage actress Mary Pickford, future president of the United States Franklin Delano Roosevelt, and then-current president Woodrow Wilson, though all of them survived.

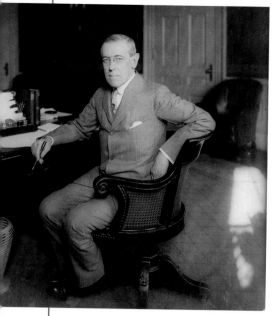

Although President Woodrow Wilson fell victim to the Spanish flu in 1919 while trying to negotiate the Treaty of Versailles to end World War I, he made a full recovery.

Genetic Components

Today, scientists know that the influenza virus that caused the pandemic came in several strains. The first strain was designated as H1N1. Another type of strain called H2N8 (which has not been seen again in the general population) was also responsible.

The genetic makeup of the influenza virus is characterized depending on two genes that interact with each other. The first (letter H) is hemagglutinin, and the second (letter N) stands for neuraminidin. The viruses are then grouped into three possible categories: influenza A, B, and C. Different subtypes develop because of mutations that create new genetic combinations. For the influenza A group, sixteen possible H subtypes and nine possible N subtypes are possible. Even more subtypes exist for groups B and C. It's important to note, however, that A and B viruses are of concern for human health, and only influenza A has the potential to cause pandemics.

Asian Flu

Influenza may have caused the most damage right after World War I, but more pandemics were to come as the twentieth century continued. The Asian flu, named because it was first identified in China before crossing the Pacific, caused 70,000 deaths in the United States between 1957 and 1958. When this particular virus went through a genetic mutation—changing into H3N2 (another form of influenza A)—it resulted in the Hong Kong flu, leading to more than 34,000 deaths in the United States. This occurred because the virus was first detected in Hong Kong in 1968 before moving to North American shores. This particular virus still circulates today, but its effects are much milder, leading only to seasonal flu outbreaks in isolated areas.

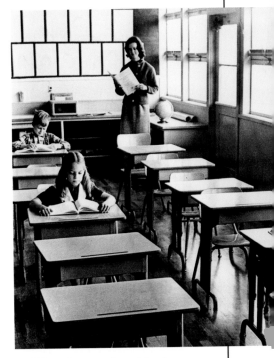

California teacher Marianne Strader looks over a nearly empty classroom as school attendance was at an all-time low in 1969 during the U.S. outbreak of Asian flu that year.

Swine Flu and Russian Flu

The 1970s saw some potential flu threats in the form of swine flu in 1976 and Russian flu in 1977.

The former, when first identified at the Fort Dix military base in New Jersey, worried experts because the virus was thought to be related to the Spanish flu virus of 1918. (As it turned out, later research demonstrated that had this flu strain spread, it would have caused much less damage than the Spanish flu had.) The latter led to many cases of the flu in persons under the age of twenty-three, but did not spread to older individuals because of the timing of the virus's appearance. The Russian flu was a strain of H1N1, which had circulated in many areas prior to 1957. Thus, persons born before 1957 were likely to have been exposed to H1N1 viruses and to have developed immunity to them. Because the Russian flu spread primarily among children, it was not considered a true pandemic.

By the 1980s and 1990s, concerns about a pandemic flu subsided, but that was only because the world was becoming more concerned about other newly emerging infectious diseases.

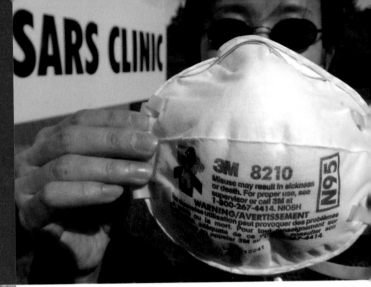

Emerging Diseases

4

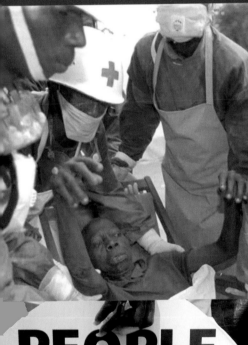

People say I can smell viruses, but I've never smelled a virus. It's more than just instinct. It's also about being interested in what is going on, having the right technique and the right people, as well as the expertise. I'll admit that a little luck and being at the right spot at the right time has something to do with my achievements, but it's also about anticipating things.

—Albert Osterhaus, Ph.D.,
New Scientist, 2005

At the moment, there are many diseases that are causing a great deal of concern in

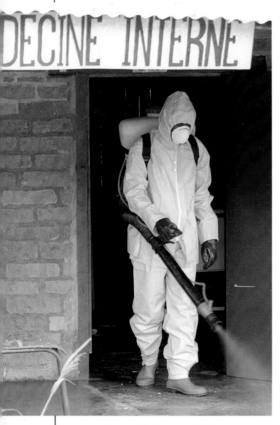

DECINE INTERNE

A member of the health department of the Gabonese army spreads disinfectant at a Mekambo hospital to prevent the spread of the Ebola virus there in 2001.

public health agencies and governments across all continents. Some of them, like Ebola, Bolivian hemorrhagic fever, and Marburg virus, are highly contagious and may have a limited ability to become pandemics. If any of these viruses became widespread, however, their effects would be unparalleled. These diseases have not developed into serious worldwide threats because they actually "burn out." In other words, they are so potent that transmission from one person to another is controlled. However, because of the nature of biology, there can be mutations in the genes that cause these diseases, potentially increasing the possibility that any of them could become more sustained and have the increasing ability to develop into a pandemic. In North America, the three diseases that present the greatest risk are HIV/AIDS (human immunodeficiency virus/acquired immunodeficiency syndrome), severe acute respiratory syndrome (SARS), and avian flu.

HIV/AIDS

In the twenty-five years since AIDS was first discovered, it has killed more than 25 million people, making it among the most destructive pandemics in history according to the World Health Organization. HIV is spread through unprotected sex, exchange of bodily fluids through blood transfusions and intravenous drug use, and transmission between mother and child.

Today, more than 40 million people around the world are living with HIV, the virus that causes AIDS,

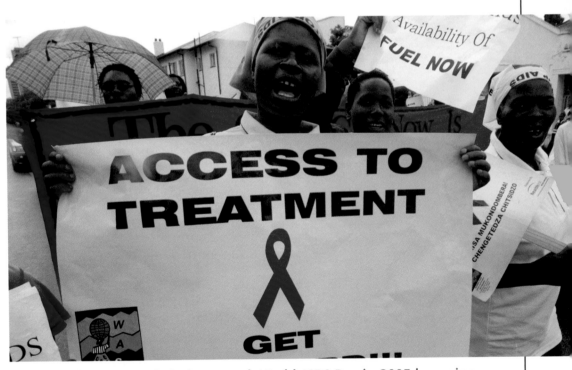

Protestors in Harare, Zimbabwe, mark World AIDS Day in 2005 by urging public health officials to offer HIV treatments for all those affected by the virus in Africa.

and there is no known cure for the disease. The Western world has significantly reduced the death rate due to AIDS with antiretroviral drugs (named because they can slow down the progress of the virus and help limit its damage to the body's immune system). In the 1980s, when the virus first appeared, this rapid reduction in the immune system's ability to fight disease was nearly an instant death sentence. But while the United States now has access to antiretroviral drugs, the story is quite different in African and other developing nations where millions currently suffer from the biological effects of the disease, as well as the social stigma associated with it. In 2005, AIDS claimed approximately 2.8 to 3.6 million people around the world, many of whom were children.

SARS

While AIDS is an ongoing problem, another pandemic with a curious beginning has quietly faded from memory. The respiratory disease called SARS first appeared in November 2002 in China's Guangdong Province when a man there reported suffering flu-like symptoms and a high fever. Over the next few months, SARS spread through Asia, Canada, the United States, and Europe, leading to 8,908 infections and 774 deaths. For much of 2003, the news was filled with stories about the spread of SARS, especially because scientists did not yet know what

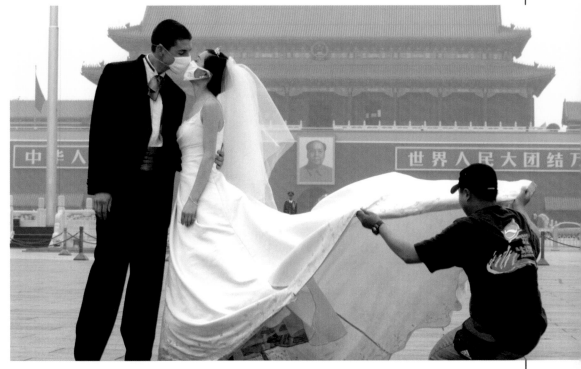

New Yorker Mathieu Borysevicz *(left)* kisses his bride Zhang Yu from Beijing, China, through facial masks to protect against the transmission of the SARS virus during an outbreak there in 2003.

the disease was and how it was spread; plus antibiotics had proved ineffective in treating it. By 2005, the *New York Times* reported that "not a single case of severe acute respiratory syndrome has been reported this year or in late 2004. In addition, the epidemic strain of SARS . . . has not been seen outside a laboratory since then."

One of the reasons for the halting of the spread of SARS was the discovery by scientists in 2003 that the coronavirus, which was detected in bats, monkeys, and cats, had caused the disease. They also sequenced its genetic code in laboratories to further understand the molecular underpinnings of SARS. A second reason SARS was contained was due to vigilant efforts to quarantine the disease by the Chinese government in alerting various health organizations. Because we have a much better idea of what to do in the event of a new SARS case, this "heightened preparedness" will prevent the rapid outbreak seen in 2003.

Avian Flu

The lessons learned from SARS may have to be applied more quickly than first thought because of continuing concerns that a new influenza pandemic is about to be unleashed. Avian (or bird) flu, which is caused by the type A influenza virus, was first identified more than a century ago in Italy, where it was confined for several decades. Even though avian flu cannot yet be categorized as a pandemic, it has been viewed as a pandemic threat since 2003, when an outbreak (which began in the Southeast Asia) took place. At the time, WHO issued a warning, reporting that this avian flu outbreak is "the largest and most severe on record. Never before in the history of this disease have so many countries been simultaneously affected, resulting in the loss of so many birds."

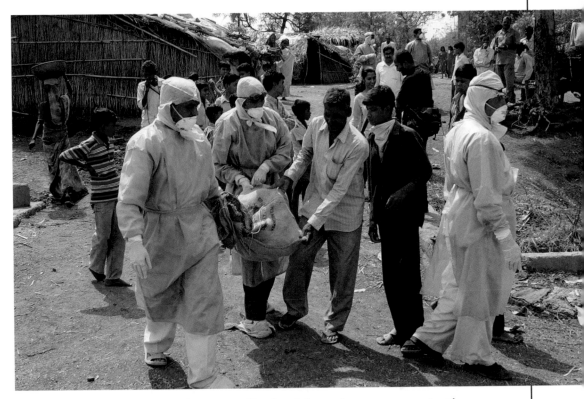

In this 2006 image from Jalgaon, India, health workers wear protective suits. They are carrying chickens to be slaughtered as a preventive measure to safeguard against the spread of avian flu.

WHO went on to say that all birds are thought to be at risk for avian flu, even though some species such as wild ducks are more resistant to the disease than others. Other types of poultry, like chickens and turkey, are also vulnerable to the onset of flu, with symptoms ranging from mild illness to a highly contagious and rapidly fatal disease, with a mortality rate nearing 100 percent.

Influenza Subtypes

Why is the rampant spread of avian flu among birds, as well as livestock and other animals, important for humans? There are several reasons for this correlation. First, there is a risk of direct infection when the virus passes from poultry to humans, resulting in very severe disease. There have been several influenza viruses that have crossed the species barrier to infect humans, including H1N1 (the cause of Spanish flu), H2N2 (Asian flu), and H3N2 (Hong Kong flu), all discussed in earlier chapters. All of these instances of influenza share a process known as antigenic shift, where one genetic portion of the virus mutates to create an entirely different genetic composition. The newer genetic version can be more effective at infecting humans.

As previously mentioned, influenza A has sixteen possible H subtypes and nine possible N subtypes, but only viruses of the H5 and H7 subtypes are known to cause the most virulent forms of the disease. When we talk about avian flu, or it is mentioned in the media, what's meant is the influenza A virus known as H5N1. This genetic version of the flu, discovered by a team of laboratory researchers in Rotterdam, Holland, led by Dr. Osterhaus, has had the greatest impact on birds and poultry since 1997. At that time, the H5N1 strain infected eighteen humans, causing six deaths. Scientists in Hong Kong discovered that all those who died had been exposed to poultry because they worked in the agriculture industry. When other people began showing signs of infection, the country's entire poultry population—estimated at around 1.5 million birds—was destroyed within three days of the first case of H5N1-strain avian flu.

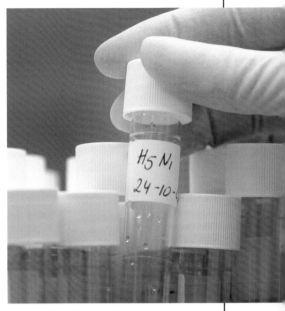

An employee of the Dutch company Intervet works on an experimental influenza vaccine for birds in 2005 to help eliminate the H5N1 virus.

Unlike typical seasonal influenza, where infection causes only mild respiratory symptoms in most people, the virus caused by H5N1 is unusually aggressive, with rapid deterioration and a high rate of fatality. Primary viral pneumonia and multi-organ failure are common. In the present outbreak, more than half of those infected with the virus have died. Most cases have occurred in previously healthy children and young adults. Since that first outbreak in Hong Kong, there have been more than 200 deaths of people in fifty countries, including Japan, Malaysia, Romania, Turkey, Vietnam, and Egypt.

Transmission

Thus far, the H5N1 strain of avian flu has largely been transmitted from bird to bird, or from bird to person, except in a 2006 case in Indonesia where a mother passed the virus onto other family members. This "cluster" of human-to-human transmission is a signal that the virus is closer to becoming capable of infection at the pandemic level, according to WHO officials. Genetic sequencing of the virus taken from those infected proved that the virus had been transmitted from one human to another, and not from the direct contact of infected poultry. Although the Indonesian case became the first documented proof of the human-to-human transmission capabilities of the H5N1 strain of influenza, WHO scientists also have strong evidence to support a similar transmission of H5N1 in a Thai family in 2004.

In all other cases of the H5N1 strain thus far, the main route of human infection is through direct contact with infected poultry, or surfaces and objects contaminated by the animals' feces. But there is an even greater concern that the virus, if given enough opportunities, will change into a form that is highly infectious for humans. The H5N1 strain is particularly worrying, says WHO, because:

- Laboratory experiments have shown that the strain mutates rapidly and seems to acquire genes from viruses infecting other animal species.
- The H5N1 strain of influenza can cause severe disease in humans, as demonstrated by its large percentage of fatalities.

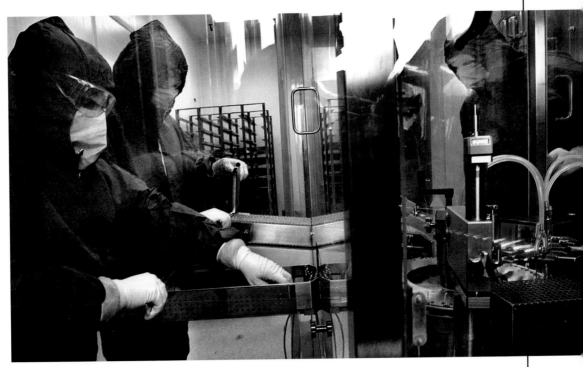

Local employees of the Hungarian company Omninvest check some vials of vaccine against the H5N1 avian flu virus in 2006.

- Birds that survive infection excrete viral germs orally and in feces, for at least ten days, helping spread the virus at live poultry markets and by migratory birds.
- The more birds infected with bird flu, the greater the opportunity for direct infection of humans.
- As more humans become infected, the greater the likelihood the virus will mutate into one that spreads easily between humans, and not only from the result of contact with infected poultry or their feces.

If the H5N1 strain follows this plan, then it could become the next source of a major global pandemic. But this assumes that the mutation of the virus occurs extremely quickly, which some scientists claim is unlikely. Another, more gradual mutation could take place in a process called adaptive mutation, where the ability of the virus to infect humans increases in a way that is directly related to the overall increase in human infections. In other words, the more opportunity the virus has to infect humans, the worse the infection becomes. But these infections would likely be transmitted in small clusters over a period of time instead of within large groups quickly, thus allowing emergency plans to be implemented to hopefully avert a potential pandemic, or at least better control one if it occurs.

There is no question that the risk of human-to-human transmission of the H5N1 strain is very serious, and that more cases of avian flu in humans increase the likelihood that a pandemic could occur. Only a small number of genetic mutations need to take place for the H5N1 flu to become a pandemic virus like the one of 1918. Despite the risk, new technologies are being developed and new treatments are being tested to halt the potential progress of avian flu.

ew Technologies and Treatments

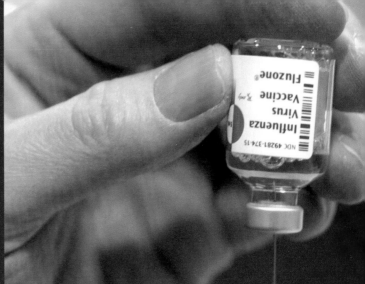

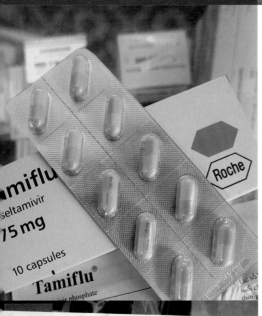

amiflu
seltamivir
75 mg
10 capsules
Tamiflu®
hosphate

Roche

u Clinic
arts at
:00 pm
 Clínica para
uenza empieza
hoy a las
3:00 pm

Flu Shot
Line
forms in
the rear of
Building

At the moment, much of what we know about what drugs could be used to treat a pandemic flu is based on the knowledge we have from the effects of the Spanish flu nearly a century ago. This information may not be very useful because of the information-gathering abilities of that time. As a result, much research has occurred in trying to determine what would be the best possible course of action to take when treating a pandemic flu, or to prevent it entirely. Several classes of drugs, including antibiotics,

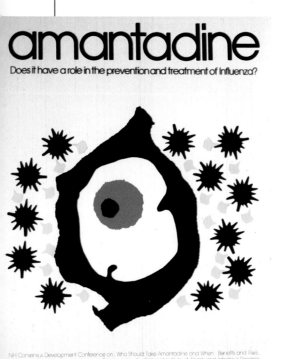

amantadine

Does it have a role in the prevention and treatment of influenza?

NIH Consensus Development Conference on: Who Should Take Amantadine and When. Benefits and Risks and Use in Combination with Vaccines. Sponsored by the National Institute of Allergy and Infectious Diseases

October 15, 1979, Masur Auditorium, NIH Bethesda, Maryland 20205. For information Call John LaMontagne 496-7051

This poster for a 1979 conference for representatives of the National Institute of Health (NIH) advertises the influenza drug amantadine.

antivirals, and vaccines, have since been developed in the last three decades, each with varying effects that may or may not be useful to slow or limit the spread of influenza.

Drug Treatments

Antiviral drugs are used to treat viral infections. They are best known for treating immune-suppressing diseases such as HIV, herpes, and hepatitis B and C, but they can also be used to treat specific strains of influenza. These drugs work in various ways to combat the virus. For example, an antiviral drug can attack when the virus attaches itself to the host cell, when the virus replicates inside the host (human), or when viral components are assembling themselves to become full viruses.

In the case of the flu, one particular drug, amantadine (commercially known as Symmetrel), quickly became the standard for treating influenza A after it received approval in 1976 by the U.S. Food and Drug Administration (FDA).

Amantadine works because it interferes with a viral protein, M2, which is required for the virus to become "uncoated" once it is taken inside the cell. But because the drug was previously used in China to protect its birds against the onset of avian flu (2.6 billion estimated doses of amantadine were administered), it meant that the H5N1 strain originating from Southeast Asia is most likely resistant to treatment by amantadine. As a result, the CDC has recommended that amantadine not be prescribed in future flu seasons, increasing the likelihood that it may one day become effective for influenza prevention in humans should a pandemic of influenza A arise.

A derivative of amantadine (rimantandine) can also be used to treat influenza A. Approved in 1994, scientists don't really know why this drug works. They believe that the virus M2 protein may play a role in decreasing the flu virus's ability to replicate inside the human body and infect other humans. However, rimantadine suffers from the same resistance issues as its parent drug, and so it may not be effective for pandemic flu either.

More recently, another class of drugs that acts on the neuramidase (or N) portion of the influenza virus has shown some promise for treating the flu. These drugs, specifically oseltamivir (commercially known as Tamiflu) and zanamivir (commercially known as Relenza) work by preventing new viruses from emerging from infected cells, which can then reduce the severity and duration of typical seasonal influenza. The effectiveness of these drugs depends on them being administered within forty-eight hours of the onset of flu symptoms. Another advantage these drugs have is that they work on a wide variety of flu strains because the genetic sequence that is specifically targeted is almost the same in any seasonal flu virus.

Are We Ready?

The most obvious question remains: Would Tamiflu and Relenza work in the event of a massive pandemic of H5N1 influenza? One study suggested that higher doses and longer durations of therapy with Tamiflu could be used for the treatment of patients with H5N1, though scientists are uncertain about the reliability of the drug to prevent human-to-human transmission of the virus. So, while H5N1 is much less likely to be resistant to Tamiflu, the same study also found that the standard recommended dose of Tamiflu (75 mg twice daily for five days) does not fully suppress the virus's ability to spread rapidly in patients. In a related study, Relenza was also found to reduce flu symptoms if taken within forty-eight hours of the onset of symptoms.

The United States and many other countries are stockpiling Tamiflu and Relenza for use in the event of a pandemic, but these drugs are more expensive to produce than amantadine, which is readily available.

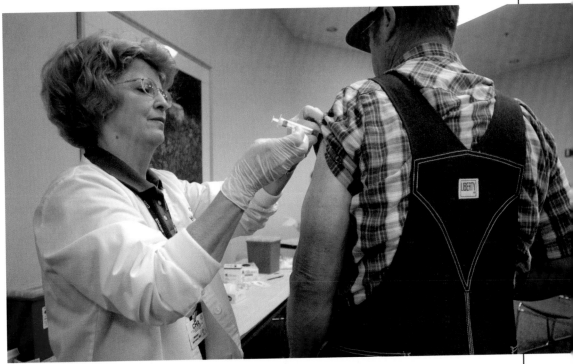

Nurse Wanda Norman gives a flu shot to Fred H. Wallace at a health center in Kannapolis, North Carolina, in 2004, a year in which there was a shortage of influenza vaccine.

They are also in limited supply. There is a particular delay in producing Tamiflu, according to the drug's parent company, Roche, because of the availability of shikimic acid. This acid is expensive to produce and is only effectively isolated from Chinese star anise, an ancient cooking spice. Ninety percent of the star anise harvest is currently used by Roche in making Tamiflu.

Although scientists downplay the importance of how to produce shikimic acid, it doesn't change the fact that making Tamiflu is a very complex, multi-step process involving several chemical reactions. Increasing the production volume would require construction of extensive new facilities and a minimum of six months to acquire all of the materials needed. Large quantities of Tamiflu were stockpiled beginning in 2005, and even though these quantities number in the millions of doses, the amount is still insufficient to protect large populations.

Influenza Genome Sequencing Project

Because understanding the underlying genetic basis of flu strains is so important in predicting how the virus will affect people, a new government initiative was created to sequence genetic codes and link them to potentially lethal strains. The Influenza Genome Sequencing Project (which is funded by the National Institute of Allergy and Infectious Diseases) is, according to its Web site, a collaborative effort designed to increase the genome knowledge base of influenza and help researchers understand how flu viruses evolve, spread, and cause disease. The project hopes that by making available as many genetic sequences of flu strains as possible, new vaccines, therapies, and diagnostics can be developed and will improve what we know about how influenza pandemics emerge. As of January 2006, 684 isolates have been completely sequenced from avian flu viruses known to be present in human populations.

GIS Technology

Another method of tracking where avian flu may take place is the use of geographic information system (GIS) technology, which is one of the most powerful weapons available to track the spread of disease, according to Sherrill Davidson, associate professor of avian medicine and pathology at the University of Pennsylvania. Since 1998, scientists at the university have been using GIS to map the location of commercial poultry flocks, feed

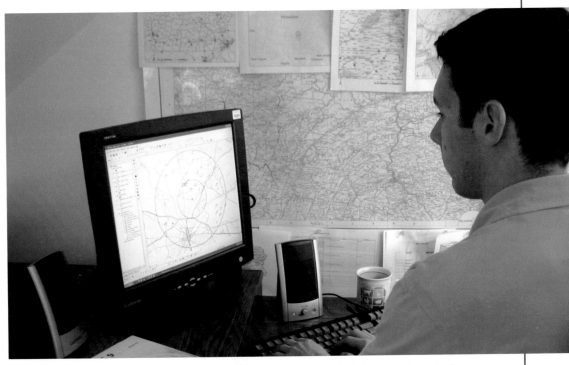

In this photograph from the Laboratory of Avian Medicine and Pathology in Pennsylvania, a technician uses geographic information system (GIS) technology to help monitor disease outbreak.

mills, processing plants, rendering plants, hatcheries, and components of the live-bird market system through-out the Commonwealth.

The New York State Department of Health also has GIS technology available, but to date it has only used it to track potential bioterrorism agents and the West Nile virus, which, while not a pandemic, has led to the deaths of several hundred people over the last decade.

A new and particularly exciting development is taking place, thanks to the capabilities of the Internet. Google Earth was originally built using government satellite imagery to map major outposts of the world, but its applications go much further. Aside from being able to locate people's houses and major landmarks, it can also be used to map where influenza outbreaks have occurred. Declan Butler, the European correspon-dent for *Nature*, has created a map that is updated with the latest information as to where a new instance of avian flu has developed. He has already mapped 2,500 outbreaks from a two-year period, which also show all confirmed human cases of infection with the H5N1 influenza virus in the same period. This map could be a powerful tool in predicting where future influenza out-breaks may take place, crucial information that could help save lives during a pandemic.

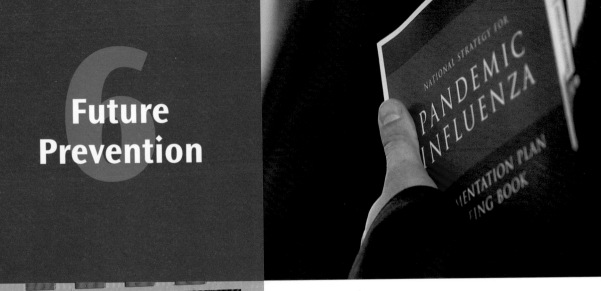

6 Future Prevention

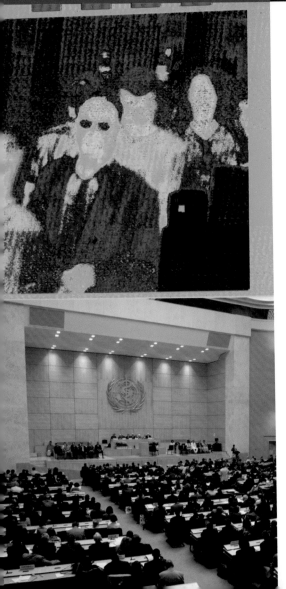

With all the information that we have about what a pandemic is, what impact could it have on the world? What can we do when a new pandemic has begun and is spreading? Are we prepared for such an event? The World Health Organization claims that we are not prepared. Representatives from WHO estimate that much more work needs to be done to battle the onset of a pandemic effectively. They also admit that it's not a matter of stopping a pandemic from

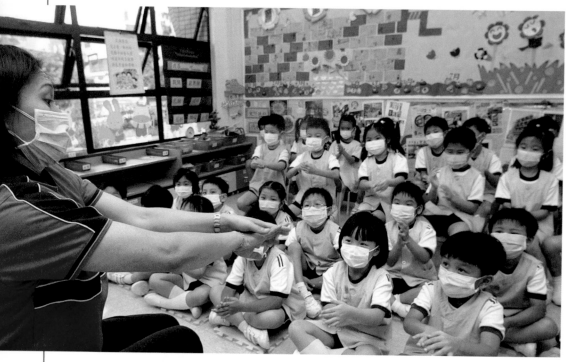

A teacher in Hong Kong illustrates to students the importance of hand washing during the first day back to school after quarantines kept public buildings closed during the SARS epidemic in 2003.

happening, but perhaps delaying its arrival or minimizing its effects.

Taking Precautions

While no scientist or health organization knows with any certainty if a pandemic can be prevented, you can take precautions to help keep you, your friends, and your family healthy and safe. The first precaution is to wash your hands frequently and thoroughly with soap and water, especially after using the bathroom, before eating, and after being around someone who is sick. A second precaution for those who have pet birds is to keep the bird, and its food and water, safely away from other birds that may be infected with the flu virus. Keep the bird's cage clean, and make sure to wash your hands after touching or petting the bird.

Fortunately, many countries such as Australia, Canada, and the United States are setting specific guidelines of what to do in the event of a pandemic. Much of this containment will likely be accomplished by following official health advisory announcements. People may be instructed to remain inside their homes, avoiding large public gatherings such as stadium events, and to temporarily remain home from work or school. Other instructions could be to restrict transportation by commercial airplane or rail systems. Finally, governments could possibly isolate people in quarantines or install a curfew.

WHO has also prepared a pamphlet that lists several recommended strategic actions, which are broken down into three phases:

- **Pre-pandemic phase:** Reduce opportunities for human infection and strengthen the early warning system.
- **Emerging pandemic virus:** Contain or delay spread at the source.

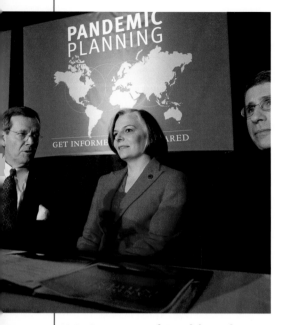

U.S. Secretary of Health and Human Services Mike Leavitt *(left)*, director of the CDC Julie Gerberding, and director of the National Institute of Allergy and Infectious Diseases Anthony Fauci speak on pandemics in Washington, D.C., in 2005.

- **Pandemic declared and spreading internationally:** Reduce morbidity, mortality, and social disruption, and conduct research to guide response measures.

    According to the U.S. government, there are several measures that could be taken in the event of a pandemic:

- Treating sick and exposed people with antiviral medication (such as Tamiflu or Relenza)
- Isolating sick people in hospitals, homes, or other facilities
- Identifying and quarantining exposed people
- Closing schools and workplaces as needed
- Canceling public events
- Restricting travel

In addition, people should protect themselves by getting seasonal flu shots, washing their hands frequently, and staying away from others who are sick.

What Will the Future Hold?

Will these measures be effective should a pandemic arise? It's impossible to know at this point, but there are differing viewpoints on whether the current measures for pandemic management and prevention are restrictive enough. Other people believe that containment tactics have the potential to be overly restrictive. Quarantines, for example, have been shown to have an uneven effect when it comes to curbing the spread of disease.

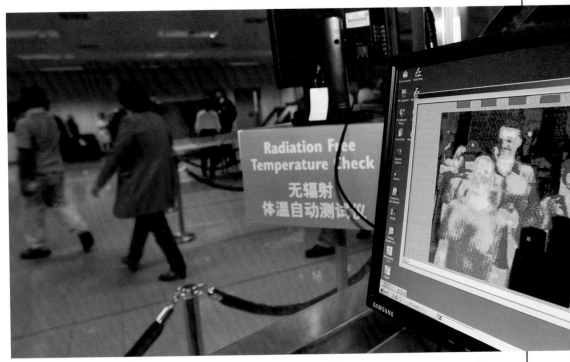

Passengers leaving Changi International Airport in Singapore pass through a thermal scanner that detects body temperatures to eliminate the chances that a person sick with SARS will spread the virus.

In China, quarantines helped limit the spread of SARS once the underlying genetic basis was identified and could be traced almost exactly to the first persons who had the disease. But in the case of a potential pandemic such as the H5N1 virus, quarantines may not be enacted quickly enough to be effective.

Another important issue is that a pandemic will affect people who live in cities differently than people who live in rural areas. In a city such as New York, where many people are crowded into a small area, a disease can spread so rapidly that thousands may be affected by the end of a single day. In a rural setting, there are only a few people per square mile, so the disease has much farther to go to have the same impact.

> *. . . in the case of a potential pandemic such as the H5N1 virus, quarantines may not be enacted quickly enough to be effective.*

Ultimately, we still don't know when, or if, a pandemic may occur. Scientists are understandably worried, and governments around the world have many plans in place. The media will continue to sound alarm bells about the eventuality of a global disease outbreak. The people's response should be education and awareness—the only ways in which we can ready ourselves for new outbreaks of disease. In other words, having common sense, sound judgment, and being realistic about all possibilities is the best way to minimize the effects of a pandemic.

Glossary

AIDS (acquired immunodeficiency syndrome) An infectious, often sexually transmitted disease that ravages the immune system.

amantadine An antiviral drug used to treat the flu.

antibiotic Medication used to treat bacterial infections.

antiviral A type of drug that kills or weakens a virus, or interferes with the ability of a virus to replicate.

avian flu An influenza virus that infects birds.

bacteria Any of a large group of single-cell organisms that live in soil, water, plants, organic matter, or the live bodies of animals or people.

CDC (Centers for Disease Control and Prevention) A U.S. government agency in charge of tracking, recording, and controlling major infectious diseases.

contagious Easily spread from one person to another.

epidemic An outbreak of a contagious disease that spreads quickly and affects many people.

flu The shortened, common name for influenza.

germ An informal term for a disease-causing microorganism (bacteria or virus).

H5N1 A subtype of avian influenza virus A, which experts believe may mutate into a form that transmits easily from person to person.

hemagglutinin A substance in the blood that causes it to clot.

immune system The parts of the body that act together to protect it against infection or disease.

immunization The process of rendering a person protected (immune) against a certain disease.

infection The invasion of the body by microorganisms (such as bacteria or viruses) that cause disease.

influenza A contagious disease in which there is fever, coughing, sneezing, and muscle pain. Influenza is caused by a virus and often occurs in epidemics.

mortality rate The ratio of deaths in an area in relationship to the population of that area.

pandemic A global outbreak of infectious disease, like influenza.

pathogen Anything capable of causing disease, which usually refers to organisms such as bacteria, fungi or viruses.

quarantine The isolation of a person or group in order to contain an infectious disease's ability to spread.

re-assortment When the eight segments of a virus "mix and match" so that a new combination of the eight segments is produced.

Relenza The brand name for one of two drugs available for the treatment of avian flu.

replicate To make a copy or duplicate of something. A virus must make many copies of itself in order to spread and infect other people.

seasonal flu This is a common strain of influenza that is transmitted from person to person. Unlike avian flu, most people have some immunity to seasonal flu, and vaccines are readily available to combat it.

symptom An indication that a person has a condition or disease. Some examples of symptoms are headache, fever, fatigue, nausea, pain, and rashes.

Tamiflu The brand name for one of two drugs available for the treatment of avian flu. This drug is currently the most popular choice for flu treatment.

transmission The passing of an infectious disease from one person or group to an uninfected person or group.

vaccine A preparation of weakened microorganisms given to create or increase resistance to a certain disease. It can be administered with a needle or by mouth.

virus A microscopic structure that can grow and reproduce only by invading a living cell. Once a virus enters a cell, it can multiply and cause infection in a person or other living thing.

For More Information

Centers for Disease Control and Prevention (CDC)
1600 Clifton Road
Atlanta, GA 30333
(800) CDC-INFO (232-4636)
Web site: http://www.cdc.gov

U.S. Department of Health and Human Services
200 Independence Avenue SW
Washington, DC 20201
(877) 696-6775
Web site: http://www.hhs.gov

The World Health Organization (WHO)
525 23rd Street NW
Washington, DC 20037
(202) 974-3000
Web site: http://www.who.int

Web Sites

Due to the changing nature of Internet links, Rosen Publishing has developed an online list of Web sites related to the subject of this book. This site is updated regularly. Please use this link to access the list:

http://www.rosenlinks.com/in/pand

For Further Reading

Aronson, Virginia. *The Influenza Pandemic of 1918*. New York, NY: Chelsea House, 2000.

Barry, John M. *The Great Influenza: The Epic Story of the Deadliest Plague in History*. New York, NY: Viking Press, 2004.

Davis, Mike. *The Monster at Our Door: The Global Threat of Avian Flu*. New York, NY: The New Press, 2005.

Getz, David, and Peter McCarty. *Purple Death: The Mysterious Flu of 1918*. New York, NY: Henry Holt and Co., 2000.

Greene, Jeffrey, and Karen Moline. *The Bird Flu Pandemic: Can It Happen, Will It Happen?* New York, NY: St. Martin's Press, 2006.

Kolata, Gene. *Flu: The Story of the Great Influenza Pandemic*. New York, NY: Touchstone Books, 2001.

Peters, Stephanie True. *The 1918 Influenza Pandemic*. Tarrytown, NY: Benchmark Books/Marshall Cavendish, 2005.

Siegel, Marc. *Bird Flu: Everything You Need to Know About the Next Pandemic*. Hoboken, NJ: Wiley, 2006.

Bibliography

Biello, David J. "Ancient Athenian Plague Proves to be Typhoid." *Science News*. Retrieved April 15, 2006 (http://www.sciam.com/article.cfm?articleID= 000BF619-9B78-13D6-9B7883414B7F0135&ref= sciam&chanID=sa003).

Centers for Disease Control and Prevention. "Pandemics Influenza: Phases." CDC. Retrieved March 20, 2006 (http://www.cdc.gov/flu/ pandemic/phases.htm).

CNN.com. "What You Need to Know About Bird Flu." Retrieved March 15, 2006 (http://www.cnn.com/ 2004/WORLD/asiapcf/01/21/birdflu.facts/).

Forth, J. "Response Planning Critical to Success of Pandemic Influenza Plan." *Epi Update*. Retrieved April 15, 2006. (http://www.doh.state.fl.us/Disease_ ctrl/epi/Epi_Updates/Epi_Weekly/10-07-05.htm).

Glasser, Ronald J. "We Are Not Immune." *Harper's Magazine*. Retrieved April 20, 2006 (http:// harpers.org/WeAreNotImmune.html).

Nature.com "Avian flu timeline." *Nature*. Retrieved April 15, 2006 (http://www.nature.com/nature/focus/ avianflu/timeline.html).

Singer, P., et al. "Ethics & SARS: Learning Lessons from the Toronto Experience." The University of Toronto

Joint Centre for Bioethics. Retrieved April 15, 2006 (http://www.yorku.ca/igreene/sars.html).

World Health Organization. "Responding to the Avian Influenza Pandemic Threat: Recommended Strategic Actions." WHO. Retrieved April 1, 2006 (http:// www.who.int/csr/resources/publications/influenza/ WHO_CDS_CSR_GIP_05_8-EN.pdf).

Index

About the Author

Miriam Segall is a writer and editor who has worked on a number of initiatives and projects related to public health matters, specifically about environmental contamination, genetic toxicology, and chemical emergencies. She lives in New York City.

Photo Credits

Cover (top left) © China Photos/Getty Images; cover (top right) Rahmad/AFP/ Getty Images; cover (bottom left) © David McNew/Getty Images; cover (bottom right) Dimitar Dilkoff/AFP/Getty Images; pp. 3 (left), 35 © Sebastian D'Souza/ AFP/Getty Images; pp. 3 (right), 45 © David Turner/Getty Images; pp. 4 (top), 5 © Mario Tama/Getty Images; pp. 4 (middle), 29 (top) © Don MacKinnon/Getty Images; p. 4 (bottom) © Christopher Furlong/Getty Images; p. 7 © Underwood & Underwood/Corbis; pp. 11, 13 (bottom), 15 CDC; p. 12 © Fabrice Coffrini/AFP/ Getty Images; p. 13 (top) © Abdulkadir Musse/AFP/Getty Images; p. 13 (middle) © Bob Bryant/Keystone/Getty Images; p. 14 Scala/Art Resource, NY; p. 16 CDC/ Courtesy of Larry Stauffer, Oregon Public Health Laboratory; p. 18 Bibliothèque Nationale, Paris, France, Archives Charmet/The Bridgeman Art Library; pp. 19, 42 Courtesy of The National Library of Medicine; pp. 21 (top), 27 © Bettmann/ Corbis; p. 21 (middle) © Scott A. Miller/Getty Images; p. 21 (bottom) © Barry Williams/Getty Images; p. 23 Musée Pasteur, Institut Pasteur, Paris, France, Archives Charmet/The Bridgeman Art Library; p. 24 Courtesy of the National Museum of Health and Medicine, Armed Forces Institute of Pathology, Washington, D.C. (NCP 1603); p. 26 Library of Congress Prints and Photographs Division; p. 29 (middle) © Pool/AFP/Getty Images; p. 29 (bottom) © Don Emmert/ AFP/Getty Images; p. 30 © Desirey Minkoh/AFP/Getty Images; p. 31 © STR/AFP/ Getty Images; p. 33 © Reuters/Corbis; p. 37 © Lex Van Lieshout/AFP/Getty Images; p. 39 © Attila Kisbenedek/AFP/Getty Images; p. 41 (top) © Mike Simons/ Getty Images; p. 41 (middle) © Hoang Dinh Nam/AFP/Getty Images; p. 41 (bottom) © Scott Olson/Getty Images; p. 47 © Laboratory of Avian Medicine and Pathology, School of Veterinary Medicine, University of Pennsylvania; p. 49 (top) © Jim Watson/AFP/Getty Images; pp. 49 (middle), 53 © Paula Bronstein/ Getty Images; p. 49 (bottom) © WHO/Peter Williams; p. 50 ©Thomas Cheng/ AFP/Getty Images; p. 52 © Alex Wong/Getty Images.

Designer: Thomas Forget; Editor: Joann Jovinelly
Photo Researcher: Amy Feinberg